DEFEATING MIGRAINES WITH EXPERT GUIDANCE

Ultimate Solution Handbook For Patients, Guardians Or Family To Understand, Manage, Treat, Prevent, Reverse Symptoms And Live Well

DR. POTTER WHITLEY

has no connection to, endorsement from, or recommendation for these organizations. The author's approval or validation is not implied by the inclusion of these references.

Any direct, indirect, incidental, special, or consequential damages resulting from using or not being able to use the material in this book are not covered by the author's liability policy. For medical advice and counsel particular to their circumstances, readers are advised to check with experienced healthcare specialists.

The content, materials, and information in this book are subject to change at any time without prior notice, at the author's discretion. The text may contain errors or omissions for which the author is not responsible.

By reading this book, you understand and accept the conditions of this disclaimer.

THE REASON BEHIND THIS BOOK

For anyone facing the crippling difficulties caused by migraines, "Defeating MIGRAINES With Expert Guidance" is a source of empowerment and information. The first section of this thorough book delves deeply into the nuances of migraines, defining them and describing their different types, causes, and typical symptoms. The extensive effects that migraines can have on day-to-day functioning and general well-being are explored with the readers under guidance.

This book deftly covers the diagnosis and medical evaluation domains, emphasizing the need for expert assistance, the variety of diagnostic procedures that are accessible, and the crucial task of recognizing migraine patterns. Incorporating coexisting diseases and differential diagnoses offers more sophisticated knowledge that is essential for efficient management.

In the third chapter of this book, the scientific foundation of migraines is explored, with an emphasis on the neurological basis, the involvement of neurotransmitters, heredity, and aura. The following chapters explore various therapeutic possibilities, ranging from drugs and therapies to new technologies, building on this scientific foundation.

In chapter five, lifestyle changes are highlighted, with a focus on identifying and avoiding triggers, creating regular sleep schedules, paying attention to nutrition, and practicing stress management. The integration of holistic methods such as herbal treatments, physical activity, mind-body techniques, and supportive surroundings is advocated as essential elements of a comprehensive approach to migraine management.

This book skillfully weaves cognitive-behavioral coping methods throughout, emphasizing the contribution of cognitive-behavioral therapy (CBT) to migraine management, coping mechanism building, and emotional well-being enhancement.

This book is noteworthy for its ability to reach a wider audience by covering topics such as migraines in children, migraines during pregnancy and menopause, migraines peculiar to a certain gender, and migraines' effects on scholastic and professional lives. It offers guidance on how to go around in social and professional settings, as well as communication techniques, migraine-friendly setting creation ideas, sustaining social ties, and advocacy activities.

The examination of upcoming developments and research in migraine treatment in "Defeating MIGRAINES With Expert Guidance" demonstrates the book's forward-thinking viewpoint. This narrative looks forward, incorporating ongoing research projects, possible discoveries, technology improvements, and the critical role that patient participation in clinical trials plays.

The book reaches its zenith in the eleventh chapter, where readers are given the ability to create a customized migraine treatment plan. The construction of holistic lifestyle programs in conjunction with healthcare practitioners, ongoing monitoring, and acknowledging accomplishments highlight this book's dedication to long-term well-being.

"Defeating MIGRAINES With Expert Guidance" is essentially a more comprehensive and entertaining guide to understanding, treating, and eventually conquering migraines than your average medical manual. This book is more than just a reference; it's a travel companion that offers professional advice with compassion and uplift to help one escape the confines of a migraine.

TABLE OF CONTENT

CHAPTER ONE

AN OVERVIEW OF MIGRAINES
Migraine Definition And Types:

Intense, pulsating headaches are the hallmark of migraines, which are crippling neurological conditions frequently accompanied by other symptoms like light and sound sensitivity and nausea. An individual's everyday life is greatly impacted by these headaches, which usually linger for hours or days. While there are many different kinds of migraines, migraine with aura and migraine without aura are the two primary forms. Aura-associated migraines include visual or sensory abnormalities, such as light flashes or tingling, that occur before the headache. Conversely, migraine without aura does not present with these warning indications.

Migraines can be further classified according to factors including frequency, duration, and particular symptoms in addition to these main categories. A person's general quality of life is negatively impacted by chronic migraines, which are defined as headaches that occur on 15 or more days per month. Comprehending the subtleties associated with various migraine varieties is essential to formulating efficacious treatment plans customized to the individual circumstances of every patient.

Reasons and Inducers:

Though their precise etiology is still unknown, migraines are thought to be caused by a confluence of neurological, environmental, and hereditary variables. Given that those with a family history of migraines are more prone to suffer from them, genetic predisposition is important. Migraines can also result from anomalies in the nervous system, such as imbalances in neurotransmitters like serotonin.

Migraine attacks can be triggered by both internal and external factors. Hormonal changes can be internal triggers, particularly for women going through menstruation or a pregnancy. A wide range of things can operate as external triggers, including foods (including chocolate, coffee, and aged cheeses), sleep deprivation, stress, and environmental cues like strong smells or bright lights. To empower people to lessen the frequency and intensity of their headaches, identifying and controlling these triggers is a crucial part of managing migraines.

Typical Symptoms and Alert Signs:

Beyond just the typical headache, migraines can cause a wide range of symptoms. Frequent signs and symptoms include light, sound, and smell sensitivity, nausea, vomiting, and throbbing or pulsating pain on one side of the brain. Aura, which some people feel before the headache, might include sensory symptoms like tingling in the hands or face or visual disruptions like flashing lights or zigzag patterns.

It is essential to identify warning signals to take prompt action. Although these indicators can differ from person to person, they frequently involve minute adjustments to mood or energy levels or the beginning of particular physical symptoms hours or days before the headache happens. By keeping an eye out for and comprehending these warning indicators, people can take preventative action to lessen the severity of an imminent migraine attack.

Effects on Well-Being and Everyday Life:

Beyond the mere duration of the headache, migraines have a significant impact on everyday functioning and general well-being. Because migraine attacks are erratic, they might interfere with social interactions, employment, and personal relationships. One's involvement in different elements of life may be limited as a result of lifestyle alterations brought on by the need to control symptoms and stay away from triggers.

In particular, chronic migraines worsen emotional and mental health and set off a vicious cycle of impairment. The continual fear of having a headache can exacerbate anxiety and sadness, which in turn increases the intensity and frequency of migraines. Sleep disorders can result in a vicious cycle of exhaustion that exacerbates the difficulties migraine sufferers have.

Developing comprehensive strategies to manage and mitigate the challenges posed by this complex neurological disorder requires an understanding of the multifaceted aspects of migraines, including their definition, types, causes, triggers, symptoms, and pervasive impact on daily life. Improving general well-being and attaining better results in the face of migraines need arming people with information about their illness.

CHAPTER TWO

DIAGNOSIS AND MEDICAL EVALUATION
Seeking Expert Assistance:

Seeking expert assistance becomes essential for successful management and alleviation when dealing with the incapacitating consequences of migraines. For a precise diagnosis and customized treatment plan, it is essential to consult a healthcare expert, ideally a neurologist or headache specialist. These professionals are skilled in differentiating betwccn migraines and other headache kinds and guarantee a thorough comprehension of each person's particular migraine profile.

A comprehensive assessment of the patient's medical history is usually the first step in the diagnostic process. This entails determining probable triggers and related symptoms in addition to investigating the frequency, length, and severity of migraine attacks.

Any family history of migraines or associated neurological disorders will also be taken into account. This thorough evaluation underpins additional research and facilitates the development of a treatment plan that is customized to meet the individual requirements of the patient.

Getting professional assistance does more than only ease symptoms; it also gives people the understanding that migraines are complex conditions. Medical practitioners investigate lifestyle choices, stressors, and environmental factors that may be linked to migraine episodes. By maintaining open lines of communication, patients can take an active role in their care and offer insightful feedback that helps to improve the efficacy of later interventions and direct the diagnostic process.

Seeking expert assistance is essentially a collaborative journey towards a better knowledge and management of migraines, rather than merely a means of receiving a diagnosis. To support continued treatment and the quest for an enhanced quality of life, it forms a partnership between the patient and their healthcare professional.

Diagnostic procedures and medical tests:

Healthcare practitioners frequently use a variety of diagnostic techniques and medical tests to sort through the intricacies of migraines and create a customized treatment strategy. Although the primary diagnostic criteria for migraines are clinical symptoms and medical history, further testing may be used to further narrow the diagnosis and rule out other underlying diseases.

To rule out secondary causes of headaches, such as tumors or structural abnormalities, neuroimaging techniques, such as computed tomography (CT) scans and magnetic resonance imaging (MRI), are frequently used. With the use of these imaging methods, medical practitioners can examine the brain in great detail and detect any abnormalities or structural changes.

To examine cerebrospinal fluid for indications of infections or other anomalies, lumbar punctures, also known as spinal taps, may be advised in specific circumstances. These operations, however, are usually saved for situations in which particular worries regarding secondary headache causes exist.

It is crucial to remember that although diagnostic tests are useful instruments, they are not sufficient in the diagnosis of migraines. A complete picture of the patient's condition is ensured by a combination of a detailed clinical evaluation, a review of the patient's medical history, and, if required, focused diagnostic testing. Healthcare providers are guided by this integrated approach as they create a complex and individualized treatment plan that addresses the particular features of each patient's migraines.

Recognizing Patterns in Migraines:

To create a successful management plan that is customized to each patient's unique requirements, it is essential to comprehend and recognize migraine patterns. The frequency, severity, and presence of distinct premonitory symptoms are only a few of the many patterns that migraines frequently display.

A thorough headache journal must be kept to track migraine patterns. Important details including the beginning, length, and features of every migraine attack are documented in this journal, which is usually put together over a few weeks or months. Furthermore, variables such as possible triggers, concomitant symptoms, and reactions to certain therapies are recorded. This thorough documentation is a useful tool for medical consultations, giving medical experts a thorough picture of migraine sufferers' experiences.

It is equally vital to recognize the prodromal phase, which is marked by mild warning signals before the onset of a migraine. Mood swings, food cravings, and low energy are a few examples of these warning indicators. People can reduce the severity of an upcoming migraine episode by being proactive and recognizing these early warning signs.

Moreover, identifying the triggers that initiate migraine attacks is an essential component of pattern recognition. Environmental variables, specific foods, stress, and hormone changes are all common triggers. People can lessen the frequency and intensity of migraines by identifying these causes and making educated lifestyle changes.

Essentially, being able to recognize migraine patterns gives people the ability to take an active role in their treatment. For individuals coping with migraine issues, this individualized approach improves the accuracy of therapeutic interventions and promotes a feeling of control and a higher quality of life.

Differential Diagnoses and Concurrent Disorders:

When diagnosing migraines, a thorough and precise medical evaluation must take comorbid diseases and differential diagnoses into account. Since migraines exhibit symptoms in common with several other headache illnesses and neurological conditions, a comprehensive investigation is necessary to rule out other possible causes of the symptoms as they manifest.

Tension-type headaches are a prevalent headache type that may appear with symptoms similar to those of migraines, making them a main concern in the differential diagnosis. Making the distinction between the two is essential to creating a treatment plan that works. Healthcare providers also need to be careful to rule out secondary headaches, as these can be signs of underlying conditions including brain lesions, vascular abnormalities, or infections.

In the diagnostic process, coexisting conditions should also be taken into account. Migraine burden is increased when co-occurring conditions such as depression, anxiety, and sleep difficulties occur regularly. Since they have a substantial impact on treatment efficacy and overall quality of life, identifying and treating these comorbidities is essential to holistic migraine therapy.

Hormonal variables should also be taken into account, especially when menstrual migraines or migraines linked to hormonal swings are involved. A thorough treatment plan is developed by taking into account all relevant elements, which is ensured by this sophisticated approach to diagnosis.

In summary, a discriminating approach is necessary to navigate the terrain of migraines, taking into account not only the unique features of the headaches but also possible alternate diagnoses and comorbid diseases. This in-depth investigation guarantees the accuracy of the diagnosis and that the ensuing treatment plan takes into account the complex character of migraines, hence increasing the possibility of effective management and better patient results.

CHAPTER THREE

THE SCIENCE OF HEADACHE
Migraine's Neurological Basis:

Complex neurological processes are the cause of migraines, which are frequently incapacitating headaches accompanied by sensory abnormalities. A major factor in the development of migraines is the brain, an intricate organ. The principal mechanism entails aberrant brain activity, whereby the trigeminal nerve releases neuropeptides that induce vasodilation and inflammation. The throbbing pain that is typical of migraines is the consequence of this.

During a migraine attack, changes occur in the cerebral cortex, which is in charge of processing sensory data. Changes in blood flow have been found in studies employing cutting-edge imaging techniques, which suggest impaired brain function. Furthermore, the brainstem's involvement adds to the complexity of migraines' neurological foundation. Serotonin abnormalities in particular are responsible for the start and continuation of these neurological storms.

Developing successful therapies requires an understanding of the neurological causes of migraines. Finding certain brain areas linked to the pathogenesis of migraines presents a viable option for focused treatment. The complexity of the brain during migraine attacks is being further unveiled by advances in neuroimaging technologies, opening the door to more individualized and accurate treatment approaches.

The Genetic Predisposition to Migraine:

A significant factor in the intricate pattern of migraine predisposition is genetics. The inherited nature of migraines is evident, even though environmental variables also play a role. Research conducted on families with a history of migraines indicates a strong genetic component, with a larger chance of individuals inheriting a predisposition to these incapacitating headaches.

There are other genetic variables at work, as migraine risk is associated with several genes. The modulation of neurotransmitters such as serotonin is notably affected by specific gene variants, supporting the link between migraine neurological characteristics and genetics. Certain genetic markers linked to migraines have been identified, which offers important information about possible treatment targets.

The complex interactions between genes and environmental variables have been clarified by identifying particular genetic loci linked to migraines through genome-wide association studies. In addition to helping to understand the heredity of migraines, the identification of these genetic connections may lead to the development of more individualized treatments depending on a person's genetic composition.

Transmitters and the Chemistry of the Brain:

The beginning and development of migraines are significantly influenced by neurotransmitters, which are the nervous system's chemical messengers.

The neurotransmitter serotonin plays a crucial part in the pathophysiology of migraines. It has many diverse functions in the brain. Dilation of blood vessels, which causes the pounding pain typical of migraines, is a result of fluctuations in serotonin levels.

Another neurotransmitter that affects the onset of migraines is dopamine. Dopaminergic dysregulation has been connected to migraines, suggesting more complex brain chemistry involved in this neurological condition. The complex equilibrium that is upset during a migraine is influenced by GABA, glutamate, and other neurotransmitters, emphasizing the multifactorial character of migraines.

There is a window of opportunity for targeted therapies when the complex dance of neurotransmitters during migraines is understood. Serotonin receptor-modulating drugs, for example, work to correct the imbalance and reduce migraine symptoms. Novel pharmacological targets within the complex landscape of brain chemistry are being explored by neuropharmacologists, and this holds promise for more individualized and effective migraine treatments.

Recognizing the Significance of Aura:

The mystery surrounding migraines is further compounded by aura, a unique phase that either precedes or follows some migraines. A unique window into the underlying brain processes, the aura phase is characterized by visual disturbances, sensory alterations, and even movement symptoms.

Deciphering aura is essential to understanding migraine complexity.

Cortical spreading depression, a wave of neuronal excitation followed by inhibition, is the cause of the visual manifestations of aura, which are frequently described as shimmering lights or zigzag patterns. This occurrence adds to the series of circumstances that result in migraine discomfort and associated symptoms. Aura is an invaluable diagnostic aid that gives medical professionals vital information on the type of migraines that patients are suffering from.

Aura is significant in ways that go beyond its ability to diagnose. Treatment choices are influenced by the particular symptoms of aura, which provide information about the brain areas and circuits that are impacted. Aiming to disrupt or modify these processes, tailored therapeutics for migraine pathophysiology are made possible by the expanding understanding of cortical spreading depression that arises from studying aura.

Finally, by elucidating the neurological foundation, genetic background, neurotransmitter dynamics, and the role of aura in migraines, we can better understand these intricate headaches. This comprehensive method advances our understanding and may be the key to creating more individualized and successful migraine-fighting techniques.

CHAPTER FOUR

MEDICATION AND THERAPY OPTIONS FOR TREATMENT Prescription Drugs And Over-The-Counter Drugs

There is a wide range of over-the-counter (OTC) and prescription drugs that provide different degrees of migraine relief when it comes to managing migraines.

Those who experience lesser attacks frequently use over-the-counter medications such as acetaminophen or ibuprofen. Prescription drugs become essential, though, for migraines that are more severe or regular.

For example, triptans are a class of medications created especially to target migraines by narrowing blood vessels and obstructing the brain's pain pathways. Furthermore, ergotamine-containing drugs may also work in some circumstances, although they are less frequently recommended due to possible adverse effects.

To address the typical symptoms of nausea accompanying migraines, anti-nausea drugs may be used in addition to these treatments.

The Aspects Of Preventive Medicines To Be Considered

Preventive medicine is an important part of treatment for people with chronic or incapacitating migraines. With a proactive approach to therapy, these drugs seek to lessen the frequency and intensity of migraine attacks. Often taken for this purpose are beta-blockers, anticonvulsants, and several antidepressants.

But choosing the best preventive drug necessitates giving serious thought to a person's medical background, current ailments, and possible adverse effects.

To maximize these drugs' efficacy, frequent evaluation and modifications are frequently required. Open communication between patients and healthcare professionals is crucial for customizing a treatment plan to each patient's unique needs and reactions.

Alternative Medicines (Biofeedback, Acupuncture, Etc.)

Non-pharmacological methods provide more options for managing migraines than prescription drugs. To lessen the frequency and severity of migraines, biofeedback, for instance, teaches patients how to regulate physiological processes like heart rate and muscular tension.

Through the stimulation of particular body sites, the ancient Chinese practice of acupuncture has garnered recognition for its potential to reduce migraine symptoms. Another non-pharmacological treatment that aims to lessen the burden of migraines on daily living is cognitive-behavioral therapy (CBT), which focuses on recognizing and changing unfavorable thought patterns and actions.

These strategies show how important it is to think about personalized, holistic treatment programs for people looking for complementary or alternative therapies to orthodox medicine.

New Developments And Therapies

The field of treating migraines is always changing as a result of continued research into novel therapeutic approaches and cutting-edge remedies. Monoclonal antibodies that target calcitonin gene-related peptide (CGRP), a neurotransmitter linked to migraine symptoms, have made significant progress in this area. Through injection, these antibodies seek to inhibit CGRP receptor activation, hence lowering migraine frequency and intensity.

Moreover, non-invasive methods of managing migraines can be achieved by neuromodulation devices, such as transcranial magnetic stimulation (TMS) and external trigeminal nerve stimulation (SNS), which alter brain pathways. As migraine research advances, these novel treatments may prove beneficial for those looking for fresh approaches to managing this difficult ailment.

CHAPTER FIVE

ADJUSTING LIFESTYLE TO MANAGE MIGRAINE
Finding and Staying Away from Triggers

An essential part of managing migraines effectively is recognizing and avoiding triggers. Individual differences in migraine triggers mean that this part of the therapy approach needs to be tailored to each patient. Foods (including chocolate, aged cheese, and processed meats), hormonal shifts, bright lights or loud noises, stress, and weather variations are examples of common causes.

Maintaining a thorough headache journal can be very beneficial in identifying specific triggers. Patients and healthcare providers can find patterns and possible triggers by keeping track of food consumption, sleep habits, and environmental factors before each migraine episode.

Avoidance is the next stage after identifying triggers. Lifestyle modifications, such as dietary adjustments or the incorporation of stress-reduction techniques, may be necessary for this. Reducing migraine frequency and intensity can be achieved by decreasing exposure to identified triggers, even though avoiding all triggers may be difficult. Furthermore, knowing what triggers to avoid and how to avoid them gives people the power to make wise decisions about their daily schedules and surroundings, which improves their capacity for proactive migraine attack management.

How to Create a Regular Sleep Schedule

The management of migraines is greatly aided by a regular sleep schedule. For many people, migraines can be brought on by irregular sleep patterns, inadequate sleep, or disturbances in the sleep-wake cycle. A regular sleep pattern should be prioritized, a sleep-friendly environment should be created, and before going to bed, relaxing techniques should be used. In addition to lowering the risk of migraine episodes, getting enough good sleep is beneficial for general well-being.

A more stable internal clock that is in harmony with the body's natural sleep-wake cycle is promoted by adhering to a regular sleep schedule, which helps regulate circadian rhythms. The bedroom should be kept dark, the noise level should be kept to a minimum, and the mattress should be comfortable. The quality of sleep can also be improved by practicing relaxation methods like meditation or light stretching activities before bed. A strong basis for migraine prevention and general health is provided by incorporating these routines into daily life.

Dietary Modifications and Nutritional Factors

The management of migraines is greatly aided by dietary modifications and nutritional considerations. Several foods and substances are common migraine triggers. Among these could be meals high in tyramine, coffee, artificial sweeteners, and monosodium glutamate (MSG).

The frequency and intensity of headaches can be significantly reduced for some people by implementing a migraine-friendly diet that restricts the consumption of certain trigger foods.

Keeping a healthy, well-balanced diet is crucial for migraine prevention in addition to avoiding trigger foods. Stable blood sugar levels and a decreased risk of migraines are achieved through regular meals, drinking enough water, and focusing on complete, nutrient-dense foods.

Additionally, certain dietary supplements that have demonstrated promise in the prevention of migraines, like riboflavin or magnesium, may be beneficial for certain people. Speaking with a medical expert or certified dietitian can offer individualized advice on dietary changes and nutritional tactics catered to specific requirements.

Methods of Stress Management

A holistic approach to managing migraines must include stress management. Effective stress-reduction strategies are essential since migraines can be initiated and exacerbated by chronic stress. Including mindfulness techniques like meditation and deep breathing exercises can support relaxation and help people become more resilient to stress. The frequency and intensity of migraines have also been demonstrated to decrease with regular physical activity, such as yoga or aerobic exercise.

Finding and resolving sources of stress in day-to-day living is essential in addition to these activities. Setting realistic expectations, defining boundaries, and asking friends, family, or mental health specialists for assistance are some examples of how to do this. Reframing negative thought patterns and developing coping mechanisms are two important benefits of cognitive-behavioral therapy (CBT), which is another useful strategy for controlling stress and migraine symptoms. All things considered, incorporating stress-reduction strategies into daily life not only helps prevent migraines but also improves mental and emotional health in general.

CHAPTER SIX

COMPREHENSIVE STRATEGIES FOR RELIEVING MIGRAINES
Including Mindfulness, Yoga, and Meditation in Mind-Body Practices:

Mind-body therapies, including yoga, meditation, and mindfulness exercises, are essential parts of a holistic approach to migraine treatment. By cultivating a sense of general well-being, these activities seek to create a harmonious relationship between the mind and body. These techniques are essential for both controlling and preventing migraine attacks, as stress and tension can be major causes.

With its soft physical postures and deliberate breathing techniques, yoga eases tension in the muscles and encourages relaxation. Stress is a typical precursor to migraines, therefore the emphasis on mindful movement and deep breathing helps reduce it.

The cycle of stress and worry linked to migraines can be broken by practicing mindfulness and meditation, which also teach people to concentrate on the here and now. In addition to offering instant relief during an episode, regular practice of these mind-body methods builds long-term resilience against migraine assaults.

Moreover, studies have demonstrated that these techniques have a favorable effect on the neural pathways related to pain perception. Over time, the frequency and intensity of migraines may decrease due to a more responsive and balanced neural system, which is facilitated by yoga, meditation, and mindfulness practices. People feel more in control of their lives and are better equipped to control and lessen the effects of migraines as they grow more attuned to their bodies and pressures.

The incorporation of mind-body techniques into the holistic approach to migraine therapy provides a comprehensive approach that tackles the psychological, emotional, and physical elements of migraine management. People can improve their general quality of life by developing a conscious and centered lifestyle, which makes them more capable of overcoming the obstacles presented by migraines.

The Prevention Of Migraines With Exercise Role:

One effective—and frequently disregarded—advantage of a comprehensive migraine prevention strategy is physical activity. Although the consensus may be that exercise causes migraines, several studies have shown that it can avoid these incapacitating headaches. Frequent physical activity affects hormone balance, stress management, cardiovascular health, and overall health and well-being—all of which are closely related to the occurrence of migraines.

Aerobic exercise, like jogging, cycling, or brisk walking, improves blood circulation and encourages the release of endorphins, which are the body's natural analgesics. These physiological reactions serve as a protective barrier against stress, which is a typical migraine trigger, in addition to helping to elevate mood. Exercise also has a positive impact on sleep regulation, which is another important aspect of migraine prevention. Migraine sufferers frequently experience disturbed sleep cycles, and maintaining a regular physical activity regimen might help restore a balanced sleep-wake cycle.

Exercises that emphasize flexibility and muscle strength, like yoga or Pilates, can help reduce stress and promote relaxation in addition to cardiovascular exercise. For those whose migraines are influenced by tense muscles and bad posture, these exercises are especially helpful. To experience the long-term benefits of migraine prevention, it is imperative to establish a regular exercise regimen that suits your fitness levels and preferences.

It is crucial to remember that moderation is necessary because excessive or strenuous exercise may cause migraines in certain people. Therefore, to guarantee that the advantages of exercise are maximized without unintentionally aggravating migraine symptoms, a progressive and balanced approach to physical activity, under the advice of healthcare specialists, is recommended. To put it simply, incorporating exercise into a comprehensive migraine management plan is a proactive and long-term approach to general well-being and migraine prevention.

Herbal Medicines And Complementary Therapies:

Herbal treatments and complementary therapies offer a varied and frequently individualized approach to controlling and averting migraine attacks in the context of holistic migraine therapy. As a result of their search for more all-natural and comprehensive migraine relief, more and more people are looking at complementary therapies in addition to the standard drugs.

There has been increased interest in the possible migraine-relieving effects of herbs like feverfew, butterbur, and ginger. With its anti-inflammatory and vasodilatory properties, feverfew in particular is recognized to help lessen migraine frequency and intensity. Clinical research on butterbur has had promising results, and there is evidence that it can effectively prevent migraines. Ginger is frequently thought to have the ability to reduce migraine-related symptoms because of its anti-inflammatory and anti-nausea qualities.

Alternative therapies such as acupuncture and biofeedback have shown promising results in managing migraines, in addition to herbal medications. The ancient Chinese art of acupuncture involves inserting tiny needles into predetermined body sites to encourage the flow and balance of qi. Research indicates that by altering pain pathways and encouraging relaxation, acupuncture may help lessen the frequency and intensity of migraine attacks.

On the other side, biofeedback is a mind-body method that gives people the ability to voluntarily regulate physiological processes including skin temperature, muscle tension, and heart rate. One possible non-pharmacological method of migraine management is for people to learn how to modulate these functions to lessen the physiological reactions linked to migraines.

Given that each person's response to herbal medicines and alternative therapies is unique, it is imperative to approach them with discernment. Healthcare professionals should always be consulted as they can help people navigate the many alternatives accessible to them and ensure that migraine management is both safe and effective. The holistic approach, when combined with herbal remedies and alternative therapies, gives people a more complete arsenal to address the complex nature of migraines and customize treatments to suit their requirements and preferences.

Creating A Supportive Environment:

A key component of a comprehensive strategy for migraine management is building a supportive environment, which goes beyond targeted interventions and medicines. In addition to their physical effects, migraines have a significant negative influence on a person's emotional and social well-being. Creating a network of support and creating an atmosphere that recognizes and accepts the difficulties that migraines present can greatly improve overall management and coping strategies.

Above all, it is essential to have open lines of communication both in the personal and professional domains. Building knowledge and empathy among close friends, family, and coworkers regarding migraines, their causes, and possible effects on day-to-day functioning is beneficial. When people encounter migraine episodes, this awareness can result in a more understanding and accommodating attitude, which can lessen the stress and anxiety brought on by social demands.

It takes cooperation between companies and employees to create a migraine-friendly work environment. Adjustable work hours, telecommuting choices, and perceptive managers foster a compassionate work environment that acknowledges and adapts to the erratic nature of migraines. Furthermore, giving people a place to withdraw to during an episode that is calm and dimly lit might greatly enhance their capacity to control their symptoms and heal faster.

It's critical to create a peaceful, migraine-friendly environment at home. This could entail designating a specific area for relaxing, decreasing exposure to possible triggers like loud noises or strong scents, and adding stress-relieving features like calming colors and soft lighting. It's also critical to have a regular and sufficient sleep environment because irregular sleep patterns can make migraine symptoms worse.

In addition, emotional support is essential to the comprehensive treatment of migraines. One way for people to connect with others who have experienced similar things is by joining support groups, whether they are in-person or virtual. In these networks, exchanging coping mechanisms, wisdom, and emotional support can be quite helpful in overcoming the obstacles that migraines present.

Essentially, establishing a supportive atmosphere involves a comprehensive strategy that goes beyond isolated initiatives. It entails developing comprehension, sensitivity, and realistic compromises in both personal and professional contexts. The whole impact of these incapacitating headaches can be lessened by creating a community and setting that acknowledges and attends to the special needs of people with migraines.

CHAPTER SEVEN

COGNITIVE-BEHAVIORAL COPING TECHNIQUES
Migraine Treatment using Cognitive-Behavioral Therapy (CBT):

CBT, or cognitive-behavioral therapy, is a well-known and successful method for treating a variety of illnesses, including migraines. Cognitive Behavioral Therapy (CBT) aims to comprehend and modify the beliefs, feelings, and actions linked to migraines. The cognitive component of migraine treatment entails recognizing and combating harmful thought patterns associated with migraines, such as oversimplifying or preparing for excruciating pain. Through cognitive restructuring, people can cultivate a more pragmatic and flexible perspective, thereby mitigating the psychological effects of migraines.

The behavioral aspect of cognitive behavioral therapy (CBT) for migraineurs focuses on altering actions that could trigger or exacerbate headaches. This could entail figuring out what triggers you, practicing relaxation techniques, and forming wholesome lifestyle choices. People can lessen the frequency and intensity of their migraine attacks and regain more control over their episodes by taking care of these variables. Additionally, CBT gives patients useful pain management techniques like progressive muscle relaxation and guided visualization, which improves their ability to cope with episodes.

Additionally, CBT increases self-awareness, which enables people to identify early migraine symptoms and take preventative measures. Through consistent appointments with a licensed therapist, people can investigate the intricate relationship between feelings, ideas, and actions associated with migraines. Because of their enhanced self-awareness, people are better able to actively manage their migraines, which fosters a sense of control and lessens the helplessness that is frequently connected to long-term illnesses.

In conclusion, cognitive behavioral therapy (CBT) is an all-encompassing, empirically supported treatment strategy that targets the behavioral as well as cognitive components of migraines. CBT has the potential to greatly improve the quality of life for those who suffer from migraines by enabling them to alter harmful thought patterns, behaviors, and coping mechanisms.

Building Resilience And Coping Mechanisms:

People who suffer from migraines must learn coping strategies and resilience to deal with the difficulties brought on by this chronic illness. Developing coping techniques entails learning how to manage the social, emotional, and physical components of migraines. Identifying and avoiding triggers, such as particular foods, stressful situations, or environmental elements, is a crucial coping strategy. The frequency and severity of migraine attacks can be decreased by individuals by identifying and proactively controlling triggers.

Furthermore, developing resilience is essential while dealing with persistent migraines. Cultivating resilience is learning how to overcome obstacles, adjust to changes, and preserve emotional health despite the difficulties that migraines provide. Therapeutic methods that support emotional control and stress reduction, such as journaling, mindfulness meditation, and deep breathing exercises, can aid in the development of resilience.

Having social support is essential for managing migraines. During trying times, building a network of sympathetic friends, family, and medical professionals can offer both practical and emotional support. In addition, attending counseling or support groups can provide people with the chance to talk about their experiences, learn from others' perspectives, and get support from people going through comparable difficulties.

Furthermore, cultivating a positive outlook and acknowledging the reality of having migraines are essential to building resilience and coping strategies.

This acknowledgment of the disease, while actively working to manage and lessen its impact, does not indicate resignation. People can improve their general well-being and more skillfully negotiate the challenges of living with migraines by developing resilience and coping mechanisms.

Improving Mental Wellness:

Beyond just causing physical pain, migraines have a significant emotional cost that frequently compromises a person's general emotional health. A key component of managing migraines is addressing and improving emotional well-being, and different cognitive-behavioral techniques can help with this process.

The development of mindfulness is a crucial component in improving emotional well-being. By remaining judgment-free in the present moment, mindfulness enables people to notice their thoughts and feelings without becoming overwhelmed. Mindfulness techniques, like meditation and mindful breathing, can assist people in interrupting the vicious cycle of unfavorable thoughts and feelings linked to migraines, thus fostering a stronger sense of emotional equilibrium.

Stress management is an additional crucial element. Learning practical stress-reduction strategies is essential for emotional well-being because migraines are frequently brought on by chronic stress. Stress management techniques are frequently incorporated into cognitive-behavioral therapy (CBT), which gives patients the tools to recognize stressors, question harmful beliefs, and use coping mechanisms to lower their overall stress levels.

Additionally, improving emotional well-being requires having strong emotional regulation abilities. People can develop healthy coping mechanisms for recognizing and expressing their emotions, which can help avoid the emotional strain that can lead to migraine attacks. In CBT sessions, emotional triggers may be examined, and effective coping mechanisms for emotional reactions may be developed.

In summary, improving emotional well-being in the context of migraines necessitates a multimodal strategy that includes emotional regulation, stress reduction, and mindfulness. Despite the difficulties caused by migraines, people can cultivate a more resilient emotional state and, in the end, improve their overall quality of life by incorporating these cognitive-behavioral strategies into their daily lives.

CHAPTER EIGHT

PARTICULAR POPULATIONS AFFECTED BY MIGRAINES
Childhood Migraines: Identification And Treatment

Pediatric migraineurs face particular difficulties with diagnosis and treatment. It can be difficult to identify migraine symptoms in children because they may not express their discomfort as well as adults do. Frequent headaches, nausea, and light- or sound-sensitivity are common symptoms. To diagnose migraines in children, pediatricians frequently rely on a comprehensive physical examination, a family history, and a comprehensive medical history. MRIs and CT scans are examples of imaging studies that are usually saved for cases involving unusual features or neurological abnormalities.

Migraine treatment in children requires a multidisciplinary approach. A balanced diet, consistent sleep patterns, and adequate hydration are all important lifestyle changes. When pharmacological interventions are required, the child's age and any possible adverse effects must be carefully considered in the selection process. The efficacy of non-pharmacological interventions, like biofeedback and cognitive-behavioral therapy, in treating pediatric migraines is becoming more widely acknowledged. A key component of effective management is educating the child's parents about coping mechanisms, warning signs, and triggers.

During Menopause And Pregnancy, Migraines

For women, migraines during menopause and pregnancy present unique difficulties. Some women find relief from migraines during pregnancy because of hormonal changes, but others may find that their symptoms worsen. It is a delicate task to strike a balance between the developing fetus's safety and the need for effective migraine management. During pregnancy, non-pharmacological methods like practicing relaxation techniques and sticking to a regular schedule are frequently advised. If medication is thought to be required, the advantages and disadvantages must be carefully considered.

On the other hand, menopause is associated with a major hormonal shift that may have an impact on migraine patterns. After menopause, some women may no longer suffer from migraines, while others may notice an increase in their symptoms. Menopausal women who experience migraines may find that hormone replacement therapy (HRT) helps, but using this treatment involves carefully weighing the risks to each patient's health.

Considerations Particular to Gender

Gender-specific patterns can be seen in migraines, with women more prone to them than men. The higher prevalence in women is partly explained by hormonal fluctuations, particularly those associated with the menstrual cycle. Comprehending these gender-specific factors is essential to customizing successful interventions. Monitoring menstrual cycles and determining factors linked to hormonal fluctuations can help women take preventative action. Healthcare professionals also need to think about how contraceptives affect migraine patterns, since some formulations can make symptoms worse or lessen them.

When discussing men, the emphasis frequently moves to lifestyle elements like stress, food, and sleeping habits. Research on the possible impact of testosterone levels on migraines is just getting started. Beyond biological variables, gender-specific considerations include societal and cultural elements that could impact migraine experiences and reporting.

Effects on Professional and Academic Lives

Migraines can have a substantial negative influence on one's academic and professional life, making it difficult for people who want to succeed in these fields. Students who suffer from migraines may have trouble focusing in class, being punctual, and meeting deadlines. To foster a supportive environment, educators and school administrators must provide accommodations like flexible schedules, quiet areas for rest, and tolerance for missed class time.

Workers who suffer from migraines may find it difficult to be productive and punctual at work. Employers can help create a migraine-friendly workplace by putting in place flexible policies, reducing triggers in the workplace, and encouraging a culture of understanding. Plans for managing migraines that include rest areas and communication techniques can improve a person's overall health and performance in both professional and academic contexts. To create an inclusive and supportive environment, individuals, educators, employers, and healthcare providers must work together to address the impact of migraines on academic and professional life.

CHAPTER NINE

MANAGING WORK AND SOCIAL ENVIRONMENTS
Sharing Your Migraine Problems with Coworkers and Employers

Managing migraine in the social and professional spheres requires effective communication of challenges to peers and employers. Since migraines can have a major negative influence on one's productivity, it becomes crucial to have open lines of communication to foster a supportive and understanding work environment. When addressing employers, it's critical to explain migraines' nature and highlight their potential severity and medical validity. This entails describing the wide range of symptoms, including light sensitivity, nausea, and excruciating headaches, as well as how they can interfere with day-to-day work activities.

It's also critical to be open and honest about any potential need for accommodations. This could be the opportunity for flexible work schedules, access to a private, quiet area, or the capacity to take quick breaks during especially trying times. Giving employers information about the frequency and duration of migraines is beneficial because it allows them to plan and anticipate potential disruptions. When employers are encouraged to actively participate in finding solutions, a positive atmosphere is fostered and the conversation is framed as one of collaboration rather than obstruction.

Using a similar strategy is beneficial when discussing migraine difficulties with colleagues. Since many people may not fully understand the impact of migraines, open communication helps dispel myths surrounding the condition. Colleagues will find it easier to sympathize and provide support if you share personal experiences that humanize the struggle. Furthermore, creating a network of understanding at work can help create a more accepting atmosphere where people with migraines can talk about their needs without feeling judged.

Ways To Create Workspaces That Are Migraine-Friendly

Migraine-friendly workspaces are the result of a multidisciplinary effort that takes into account the physical and cultural elements of the workplace. Physical adjustments that employers can make include adjusting lighting, providing headphones with noise cancellation, and designating quiet spaces where staff members can hide away during a migraine attack. A comfortable and encouraging work environment also benefits from ergonomic furniture and adequate ventilation.

It is crucial to cultivate a culture of empathy and adaptability in addition to providing physical accommodations. People who suffer from migraines can significantly benefit from the implementation of policies that allow for flexible working hours, remote work options, and an understanding of leave policies. It is equally important to promote open communication and de-stigmatize the condition in the workplace. Colleague education on migraines, their effects, and how each person can help create a more encouraging atmosphere is part of this.

Apart from implementing workplace modifications, individuals can proactively establish a migraine-friendly workspace of their own. To prevent eye strain and tension, this may involve taking regular breaks, staying hydrated, and using specialized tools like blue light filters on screens. Customized coping strategies, like stress management and mindfulness, can be incorporated into everyday activities to help control migraine triggers and lessen the overall effect of migraines on productivity.

Sustaining Social Relationships Despite Headaches

Because of the unpredictable nature and intensity of the condition, people with migraines frequently experience social isolation. But keeping social ties is important for general well-being and can be done with deliberate tactics. Open communication about the difficulties caused by migraines with friends and family can build understanding and support.

People who suffer from migraines can take preventative measures when organizing social events by choosing settings that are less likely to cause attacks. Practical measures include avoiding known triggers, scheduling activities during times when migraine risk is lower, and selecting quiet, well-lit spaces. Notifying friends about probable cancellations owing to migraines guarantees comprehension and avoids miscommunication.

Virtual connections provide an alternative means of maintaining social interaction during migraine attacks in the age of technology. People can engage in social interactions without the physical strain of physically attending events in person thanks to video calls and messaging platforms. Because of this adaptability, people with migraines can continue to have relationships with friends and family despite the difficulties presented by their illness.

Another way to connect socially for migraine sufferers is through support groups and online communities. Connecting with people who are aware of the effects of migraines via experiences, advice, and coping techniques can strengthen bonds between people and lessen feelings of loneliness. Prioritizing self-care and setting boundaries when needed is crucial for ensuring that social interactions enhance mental and emotional health.

Promoting And Increasing Awareness

Promoting understanding and support for migraine sufferers on a larger scale requires advocacy and education. Misconceptions and stigma surrounding migraines may arise from the lack of thorough knowledge about the condition held by many people, including peers, employers, and the general public. The goal of advocacy work is to clear up these misconceptions and establish a supportive atmosphere for people who suffer from migraines.

Working with legislators, patient advocacy groups, and medical professionals to advance migraine research, education, and better treatment access is one way that advocacy is practiced. People with migraines can help debunk myths, inform the public, and foster empathy by taking part in awareness campaigns.

A potent advocacy tool is the sharing of personal narratives and experiences via a variety of platforms, including blogs, social media, and public speaking engagements. By making the migraine experience more relatable to others, empathy and understanding are fostered. Furthermore, it promotes candid discussions about migraines, dismantling barriers and lessening the stigma attached to this frequently invisible ailment.

Advocacy in the workplace can entail collaborating with HR departments to put inclusive policies and procedures in place that cater to migraine sufferers. This entails encouraging flexible work schedules, supplying coworkers with instruction and training, and fostering an environment where the welfare of employees is given top priority.

It is imperative to advocate for greater funding and research into migraine causes and treatments on a broader societal level. This may result in greater medical knowledge, more successful therapies, and enhanced support networks for individuals impacted. Through their active involvement in advocacy campaigns, people with migraines help create a society that is more knowledgeable, understanding, and accommodating to all those dealing with the difficulties associated with this complicated illness.

CHAPTER TEN

RESEARCH AND UPCOMING TRENDS IN THE MANAGEMENT OF MIGRAINES
Current Research Projects

The field of migraine research is dynamic, with ongoing efforts to understand the complexities of this crippling illness. The scientific community is devoting a great deal of resources to comprehending the root causes, triggers, and feasible paths toward successful intervention. The genetic basis of migraines is one important area of research.

Thanks to developments in genomics, scientists have been able to pinpoint particular genetic markers linked to migraine susceptibility. Deciphering the genetic code underlying migraines opens up possibilities for tailored therapies as well as insights into the biological mechanisms at work.

A critical component of current research pertains to investigating the role of neuroinflammation in the pathophysiology of migraines. Scholars are investigating the complex interaction between the nervous and immune systems to determine the role of inflammatory processes in migraine development. By comprehending these mechanisms, new anti-inflammatory drugs that more successfully alleviate migraine symptoms may be developed.

In addition, migraine research is placing an increasing amount of focus on personalized medicine. Customizing therapy according to a patient's genetic composition, way of life, and triggers is becoming more and more popular.

This method seeks to optimize therapeutic outcomes by tailoring interventions in recognition of the variability in migraine symptoms among patients. It is hoped that as research advances, personalized medicine will establish itself as a key component of migraine treatment, offering more accurate and effective therapeutic approaches.

Prospective Developments in the Treatment of Migraine

The field of treating migraines is about to witness revolutionary developments that could open up new directions for more focused and efficient treatments. The creation of inhibitors of the calcitonin gene-related peptide (CGRP) is one of the most promising fields. These medications have demonstrated amazing effectiveness in both preventing and treating migraine symptoms. They are made to block the action of CGRP, a neuropeptide linked to migraine attacks. The possibility of developing novel and enhanced CGRP inhibitors or different strategies that target the CGRP pathway is still very high as long as research in this area is conducted.

Furthermore, new approaches to drug delivery are being investigated to improve the effectiveness of migraine therapies. Innovative delivery methods and intranasal formulations are designed to promote the quick absorption of medications to deliver relief quickly. These developments open the door for the creation of novel compounds with improved bioavailability and targeted delivery to the affected brain regions, in addition to improving the pharmacokinetics of currently available medications.

Non-invasive neuromodulation techniques are becoming more and more promising as non-pharmacological interventions for migraine management. There is hope that devices that use non-invasive vagus nerve stimulation (nVNS) or transcranial magnetic stimulation (TMS) can lessen the frequency and intensity of migraine attacks. For those who might not tolerate conventional medication therapies or would rather not use them, these methods provide non-pharmacological alternatives.

Technological Developments in Management and Monitoring

The monitoring and treatment of migraines is undergoing a technological revolution that is empowering patients and medical professionals alike. Heart rate, sleep patterns, and physical activity are just a few of the migraine-related metrics that can be tracked in real-time with wearable devices that have sensors and accelerometers built in. Personalized treatment plans are made possible by the abundance of data, which offers insightful information about unique triggers and patterns.

Furthermore, digital platforms and smartphone apps are essential in enabling patients to take an active role in the management of their migraines. These applications frequently include tools for keeping tabs on medication adherence, documenting trigger factors, and tracking symptoms. Some even use algorithms based on artificial intelligence to scan for trends and offer tailored advice on how to change one's lifestyle or make timely interventions.

To better manage migraines, telemedicine has become essential, especially when it comes to increasing access to specialized care. Through virtual consultations, patients can communicate with headache specialists from a distance, allowing for prompt interventions and lessening the need for in-person clinic visits. Additionally, telemedicine improves continuity of care by removing geographical barriers to ongoing monitoring and plan modifications.

Clinical Trial Participation by Patients

Patients are becoming more important in the advancement of migraine research, and active participation in clinical trials is becoming more and more important. Involving patients in research priorities and outcomes that reflect the lived experiences of migraine sufferers is essential, as is assessing the effectiveness of treatments.

Through the opportunity to share firsthand experiences about how migraines affect their daily lives, patients can contribute to clinical trials, giving researchers a more complete understanding of the condition. Many migraine clinical trials now include patient-reported outcomes, such as subjective symptom assessments and quality of life measures, to ensure that the patient's perspective is taken into account when assessing treatment success.

Enhancing patient participation in research involves more than just signing up for trials. To create a cooperative atmosphere where people with migraines can exchange experiences, learn about current research, and actively influence the direction of future studies, patient advocacy groups and online communities are essential. In addition to giving patients more power, this cooperative approach makes it more likely that research findings will be translated into significant advancements in migraine treatment.

In summary, a dynamic landscape in migraine management is reflected by the intersection of ongoing research initiatives, potential treatment breakthroughs, technological advancements, and active patient participation in clinical trials. Together, these components have the potential to significantly advance our knowledge of migraines and to usher in a new era of patient-centered, individualized, and efficacious approaches to treating this common and difficult neurological condition.

CHAPTER ELEVEN

CREATING A CUSTOMIZED PLAN FOR MIGRAINE TREATMENT
Working Together with Healthcare Professionals:

Forging a cooperative alliance with medical professionals is one of the fundamental tenets of developing a customized migraine treatment strategy. Since migraines are intricate neurological disorders, getting expert advice is essential to managing them effectively. To commence, seek advice from a medical professional, such as a headache specialist or neurologist, who can perform a thorough assessment of your migraine patterns, lifestyle, and medical history. You and your partner can collaborate to pinpoint migraine triggers, assess the intensity of your attacks, and investigate appropriate treatment alternatives by maintaining open and honest communication.

When it comes to prescribing drugs specifically designed to control migraine symptoms, healthcare professionals are essential. This could involve taking preventative drugs to lessen the frequency and severity of migraine attacks as well as acute drugs to ease pain during an attack. It is crucial to schedule routine check-ups with your healthcare provider to evaluate the efficacy of the recommended treatments and make any required modifications. A flexible and adaptable approach to your migraine treatment plan is ensured by being transparent about any side effects, worries, or adjustments in your migraine patterns. Working together with medical professionals creates a sense of knowledge and support that gives you the confidence to handle the complexities of migraine treatment.

Creating A Comprehensive Lifestyle Strategy:

Comprehensive migraine management necessitates a holistic lifestyle plan because migraines are influenced by many variables other than medication. This includes taking a holistic approach that takes into account lifestyle elements like exercise, stress reduction, food, and sleep. Migraine prevention can be greatly enhanced by incorporating a regular, well-balanced eating schedule and being aware of dietary triggers, such as particular foods or additives. Furthermore, regular sleep schedules and the creation of a sleep-friendly environment improve general well-being and lessen the likelihood of migraines.

A holistic lifestyle plan must include stress-reduction strategies like yoga, deep breathing exercises, and mindfulness meditation. Regular physical activity not only helps to reduce stress but also improves cardiovascular health. To ensure the sustainability of these lifestyle changes, it's imperative to customize them to your daily routine and preferences. Working together with a medical professional or a licensed therapist can offer tailored insights into lifestyle adjustments that are in line with your unique migraine triggers and patterns. A holistic lifestyle plan builds the groundwork for long-term well-being when it is incorporated into an overall migraine management strategy.

Keeping An Eye On And Modifying Your Strategy:

Because migraines are dynamic, managing them requires constant observation and adjustment. Maintaining a thorough migraine journal that records the frequency, severity, length, and possible causes of each attack gives you and your doctor useful information. By going over this data regularly, patterns can be found, making it easier to respond proactively to possible triggers and early indicators of migraine onset.

Using technology, like migraine tracking apps, in conjunction with firsthand observations can expedite the monitoring process. These apps frequently have functions like trigger tracking, medication reminders, and report generation for talks with healthcare providers. It's critical to keep lines of communication open with your healthcare provider, sharing information about the frequency of your migraines and the efficiency of the recommended therapies. This cooperative feedback loop makes it possible to promptly modify your management plan and make sure it continues to be customized to your changing requirements.

Honoring Achievements And Preserving Long-Term Health:

Acknowledging accomplishments, regardless of their magnitude, is an essential component of preserving drive and an optimistic outlook during the migraine treatment process. Celebrate victories, such as a decrease in the frequency of migraine attacks or the ability to recognize and steer clear of particular triggers. Acknowledging and applauding these successes gives you confidence in your ability to face obstacles head-on and strengthens the effectiveness of your customized management plan.

To ensure long-term well-being, one must develop a balanced, sustainable lifestyle that promotes general health. Prioritize self-care activities, such as consistent exercise, enough sleep, and stress management, in addition to migraine management, to improve your general quality of life.

Take part in joyful and fulfilling activities to help you feel resilient when facing migraine difficulties. Even in times of relative stability, routine check-ins with healthcare providers guarantee that your management plan continues to be in line with your changing health needs. You create a strong foundation for long-term migraine management and enhanced general health by acknowledging accomplishments and placing an emphasis on long-term well-being.

[89]